Table of Contents

Types of Anaemia

Anemia is a condition that develops when your red blood cell count or hemoglobin is less than normal.

The condition is often associated with being tired and weak. The reason for this is that anemia occurs when your body doesn't have ade uate healthy red blood cells. Red blood cells carry oxygen to the body's tissues.

There are different types of anemia, including, but not limited to:

Iron-deficiency anemia, which is the most common type of anemia and occurs when your blood doesn't have enough iron to produce healthy red blood cells and hemoglobin.

The World Health Organization (WHO) states that this type of anemia, which is the most common and widespread nutritional disorder in the world, largely contributes to the fact that more than 30 percent of the world's population is anemic.

Red blood cells carry oxygen to the body's tissues and remove carbon dioxide. Not having enough working red blood cells may lead to tiredness and shortness of breath.

Aplastic anemia is a blood disorder in which the body's bone marrow — the soft tissue in the center of bones — doesn't make enough healthy blood cells. Because of this, it is sometimes referred to as bone marrow failure.

While the condition is rare, each year between 600 and 900 people in the United States are diagnosed with aplastic anemia, according to the Aplastic Anemia and MDS International Foundation, although the accuracy of the epidemiological data for the United States is still being determined. In Western countries, the incidence is approximately two per million per year, and estimated to be two- to threefold higher in Asia.

The disorder affects men and women e ually, and most commonly develops in adults between ages 20 and 25, as well as those over 60, according to the National Institute of Diabetes and Digestive and Kidney Diseases.

Sickle cell anemia is an inherited blood disorder characterized by both a deficiency of healthy red blood cells and painful episodes called sickle cell crises.

The disorder is caused by a mutation in the gene that tells the body to make hemoglobin, a protein found in red blood cells that binds to oxygen in the lungs and carries it to tissues throughout the body.

As a result of the mutation, the body produces a defective form of hemoglobin called hemoglobin S, which causes red blood cells to sickle, or develop a crescent shape.

Sickle cells are stiff and sticky and tend to block blood flow in the vessels of the limbs and organs, causing pain and raising the risk for infection.

Sickle cells also have a shorter life span than normal red blood cells, leading to an overall shortage of red blood cells and, conse uently, anemia.

Pernicious anemia refers to vitamin B12 deficiency caused by autoantibodies that interfere with vitamin B12 absorption by targeting intrinsic factor (IF), gastric parietal cells, or both. This type of anemia occurs when your body cannot absorb vitamin B12, which is needed to make healthy red blood cells and to keep the nervous system working properly.

The condition can run in families and is an autoimmune condition. B12 deficiency from low intake can also mimic pernicious anemia as they both result in anemia from reduced available B12 for red blood cell creation.

At the time it was described, PA was associated with continuous worsening of symptoms and even death without an available treatment.

With proper treatment, people who have pernicious anemia can recover, feel well, and live normal lives.

Anemia of chronic disease is also sometimes called anemia of chronic inflammation or anemia of inflammation.

Anemia of inflammation and chronic disease is considered the second most common form of anemia after iron-deficiency anemia. But the exact incidence of chronic disease anemia is not known, possibly because it's underreported and often goes unrecognized.

This type of anemia occurs when a long-term medical condition affects your body's ability to produce healthy red blood cells. Underlying conditions can vary and may include chronic illnesses such as cancer, infections, kidney disease, and autoimmune and inflammatory diseases like rheumatoid arthritis or lupus. Most often, the chronic disease prevents your body from effectively using iron to create new red blood cells, even if there are normal or high levels of iron stored in the body. Treatment for certain diseases can also affect red blood cell production.

Signs and Symptoms of Anemia

Depending on the type of anemia you have, you may experience a variety of symptoms. The most common symptom of all anemias is weakness. Here are some other symptoms.

Iron deficiency anemia symptoms may be mild, but as the condition advances, can get worse and include:

- Extreme fatigue
- Weakness
- Pale skin
- Chest pain, rapid heartbeat, or shortness of breath
- Headache, dizziness, or light-headedness
- Cold hands and feet
- An inflamed or sore tongue
- Brittle nails

- Odd cravings for ice, dirt, or starch
- Loss of appetite, most often in babies and kids

Aplastic anemia symptoms may include:

- Bleeding
- Infection
- Nausea
- Skin rashes

These symptoms may be severe from the start, or gradually worsen over time.

Other symptoms include:

- Weakness
- Shortness of breath and chest pain
- Dizziness, especially after standing up from a sitting or lying position

- Headaches

- Pale skin

- Bruising or bleeding easily

- Uncontrollable bleeding

- Nosebleeds, bleeding gums, bloody stool, or heavy menstrual bleeding

- Cold feeling in your hands and feet

- Fever due to infection

- Recurring infections or flu-like symptoms

- The appearance of small red dots on the skin that indicates bleeding under the skin

- Rapid heart rate

Sickle cell anemia symptoms can develop in some children earlier than others and typically start after the fifth or sixth month of life. Common signs and symptoms include:

- Yellowish skin, known as jaundice

- Yellowish whites of the eyes, known as icterus
- Fatigue or fussiness
- Painful swelling of the hands and feet
- Fre uent infections, especially pneumonia
- Fatigue and weakness

Episodes of pain, called sickle cell crises, occur when sickled red blood cells block blood flow to the limbs and organs

Pernicious anemia may show similar symptoms to other anemias. But because it is caused by lack of absorption of vitamin B12, and similar to inade uate B12 intake in the diet, a severe deficiency in B12 may cause:

- Tingling and numbness in hands and feet
- Muscle weakness
- Loss of reflexes

- Loss of balance

- Trouble walking

- Weakened bones, leading to hip fractures

- Neurological problems, such as confusion, dementia, depression, and memory loss

- Nausea, vomiting, heartburn, abdominal bloating and gas, constipation or diarrhea, loss of appetite, and weight loss

- Enlarged liver

- Smooth, thick, red tongue

Infants who have B12 deficiency may show the following signs and symptoms:

- Poor reflexes or unusual movements like face tremors

- Difficulty feeding due to tongue and throat problems

- Irritability

- Permanent growth problems if left untreated

14

Anemia of chronic disease may cause similar signs and symptoms to other anemias, such as fatigue, pale skin, light-headedness, shortness of breath, rapid heartbeat, irritability, and chest pain.

Red blood cells play a central role in anemia.

While white blood cells fight infection and platelets help your blood clot, red blood cells carry oxygen throughout your body.

Hemoglobin is an iron-rich protein that's found in red blood cells. Hemoglobin is what makes it possible for red blood cells to take oxygen from your lungs and carry it to places throughout your body. Hemoglobin also takes carbon dioxide from different areas of your body and brings it to your lungs so your lungs can get rid of it when you exhale.

Your bone marrow, which is in your large bones, produces red blood cells. But the vitamin B12, folate, and other nutrients that we get from food are needed to produce hemoglobin and red blood cells.

If you lack these vitamins and nutrients, you can become anemic.

In addition to not having enough red blood cells, you can also become anemic if your body gets rid of red blood cells, or if, when you bleed, your body loses red blood cells more uickly than they can be replaced.

Each type of anemia is caused by something different, and each ranges from mild to severe.

Iron-deficiency anemia develops when your body doesn't have enough iron because of blood loss, consuming inade uate amounts of iron, or having a medical condition that affects your body's ability to absorb iron from the gastrointestinal tract.

Aplastic anemia is thought to be either "acquired" or "inherited," though the exact cause is not known.

Ac uired aplastic anemia, which is more common than the inherited form, may result from:

- Toxins, including benzene (a chemical sometimes used in manufacturing and chemical synthesis), pesticides, and arsenic
- Chemotherapy and radiation therapy for cancer treatment
- Various infectious diseases, including hepatitis, HIV, and Epstein-Barr virus (a type of herpesvirus), lupus, rheumatoid arthritis, or other autoimmune disorders (those in which the immune system attacks healthy cells)
- Pregnancy

- Certain drugs, including some antibiotics, immunosuppressants, and some nonsteroidal anti-inflammatory drugs (NSAIDs)
- Cancer that has spread to the bone

Causes of inherited aplastic anemia, which is rare and develops from genes that are passed down from parent to child, include:

- Fanconi anemia
- Diamond–Blackfan anemia
- Shwachman–Diamond syndrome
- Dyskeratosis congenita

Over time, severe heart issues may develop, such as arrhythmia (irregular heart beat), angina, enlarged heart, and heart failure.

While blood tests can detect low blood cell counts and the possibility of aplastic anemia, they cannot diagnose the disorder.

Diagnosis generally re uires a bone marrow biopsy in which a special needle removes a small piece of bone marrow and bone, along with blood, for examination under a microscope.

Sickle cell anemia occurs when a person inherits two sickle hemoglobin genes, one from each parent.

A person who inherits a sickle hemoglobin gene from one parent and a normal hemoglobin gene from the other parent is said to have sickle trait.

People with sickle trait generally don't have symptoms related to it, but they are at risk of developing certain medical problems, and they can pass on the sickle hemoglobin gene to their children.

Sickle cell anemia affects millions of people around the world. It's most common in people who have ancestors from sub-Saharan Africa; regions in the Western Hemisphere (South America, the Caribbean, and Central America); Saudi Arabia; India; and Mediterranean countries such as Turkey, Greece, and Italy.

In the United States, the condition affects 90,000 to 100,000 people, and mainly affects Black Americans or African Americans.

The prevalence of the gene mutation that causes sickle cell is higher in areas of the world where malaria is found. Researchers have found that having sickle cell trait offers some survival advantage against malaria.

West and Central Africa are particularly hard hit, with a form of sickle cell anemia affecting about 1 to 2 percent of all births, according to the Sickle Cell Disease Association of America.

In the United States about 70,000 to 100,000 people have sickle cell anemia, and African Americans are affected most often, with 1 out of 365 Black American babies born with sickle cell anemia, reports the National Heart, Lung, and Blood Institute (NHLBI).

Pernicious anemia occurs when the body can't absorb enough vitamin B12 from food because it lacks a protein in the stomach called intrinsic factor, caused by autoantibodies to intrinsic factor or parietal cells. If you lack intrinsic factor, there is nothing you can do to prevent pernicious anemia caused by this.

Pernicious anemia can run in families, so having family members with the condition puts you at risk.

Since people with pernicious anemia cannot effectively absorb B12, they must receive supplemental B12 through injections or very high oral doses while monitoring blood tests.

In rare cases, another form of B12-related anemia, megaloblastic anemia, occurs simply because you're not eating enough B12. In these cases, eating foods high in B12 can help the condition. Such foods include:

- Beef, liver, poultry, and fish
- Eggs and dairy products
- Soy-based drinks and veggie burgers
- Breakfast cereals with added vitamin B12

B12 deficiency can also be caused by other factors and conditions, such as infections, surgery, medicines.

Diseases such as Crohn's and celiac can also interfere with B12 absorption.

Anemia of chronic disease can be caused by the following chronic conditions:

Inflammatory diseases, which are conditions that produce an inflammatory response in the body can cause anemia of chronic disease for several reasons:

- The inflammatory response can produce cytokines, a protein that protects the body against infection and interferes with iron processing and red blood cell production.

- Inflammation can cause internal bleeding that leads to a decrease in red blood cell count.
- Inflammation of the gastrointestinal system can interfere with the body's ability to absorb iron from food.

Types of inflammatory disease known to cause anemia of chronic disease include:

- Rheumatoid arthritis (RA)
- Ulcerative colitis
- Crohn's disease
- Inflammatory bowel disease
- Lupus
- Diabetes
- Degenerative joint disease

Infectious diseases can cause anemia of chronic disease if a person's immune system's response to the infection interferes with red blood cell production.

As with inflammatory diseases, infectious diseases can cause the immune system to release cytokines, which can interfere with the body's ability to use iron to create red blood cells. Cytokines also can block the production and function of erythropoietin, a hormone produced by the kidneys that prompts a person's bone marrow to produce red blood cells.

Infectious diseases known to lead to anemia of chronic disease include:

- HIV/AIDS
- Hepatitis
- Tuberculosis
- Endocarditis (heart infection)

- Osteomyelitis (bone infection)

Kidney failure in people with kidney disease can cause anemia of chronic disease if the disease interferes with the kidneys' production of erythropoietin. Diseased kidneys also can cause the body to absorb less iron and folate, nutrients necessary to the creation of red blood cells.

People with kidney failure also might experience iron deficiency as a result of blood loss that occurs during hemodialysis.

Certain types of cancer can prompt the release of inflammatory cytokines, which interfere with erythropoietin production and creation of red blood cells by the bone marrow. These cancers include:

- Hodgkin disease

- Non-Hodgkin lymphoma

- Lung cancer

- Breast cancer

Cancer also can harm red blood cell production if it invades the bone marrow. Moreover, cancer treatments like chemotherapy and radiation therapy can lead to anemia of chronic disease if they damage the bone marrow.

How Is Anemia Diagnosed?

In order to determine if you have anemia, your doctor will most likely talk to you about your medical and family history, give you a physical exam, and perform the following tests:

Complete blood count (CBC) A CBC will reveal the number of blood cells in a blood sample. To determine if you have anemia, your doctor will look at your blood's number of red blood cells (hematocrit) and hemoglobin.

Doctors may have different target numbers, but normal adult hematocrit values tend to range from 40 percent to 52 percent for men and 35 percent to 47 percent for women. Target adult hemoglobin values are generally 14 to 18 grams per deciliter for men and 12 to 16 grams per deciliter for women.

A test that looks at size and shape of red blood cells, called a peripheral smear Your doctor may run a test to determine if your red blood cells have an unusual size, shape, and color.

Additional tests Your doctor may recommend an invasive test to gather a sample of your bone marrow if you are diagnosed with anemia. This can help determine the cause.

Prognosis of Anemia

The prognosis of anemia depends on its type.

Iron-deficiency anemia

Most people with iron-deficiency anemia will recover fully. But if the condition is not corrected, and chronic iron deficiency persists until the red cell count and hemoglobin levels get extremely low, it can be fatal.

Aplastic anemia

While prognosis varies from person to person, the condition can be short-lived for those who develop aplastic anemia because of medications, pregnancy, low-dose radiation or infectious mononucleosis. The condition can be life-threatening if it's severe and lasts a long time or if treatments are not effective.

For those who do not recover, they may receive a bone marrow transplant from a sibling or other matched donor; their prognosis is better than for those who receive a transplant from a donor unrelated to them. And the prognosis is increasingly reported to be favorable.

For older patients with ac uired aplastic anemia, when immunosuppressive therapy is the only option, about 50 percent of people will respond well to it.

People with aplastic anemia are at higher than average risk of developing leukemia.

Sickle cell anemia

While there is no cure for sickle cell anemia, treatments can help with pain management and with preventing complications.

Improved treatments have given a better outlet for people with sickle cell anemia. As little as 40 years ago, almost 15 percent of children born with sickle cell anemia died before age 2, and many more died as teens, according to the NHLBI.

Pernicious anemia

Pernicious anemia, once it manifests, will require treatment for the duration of one's life, yet treatment is well tolerated and the disorder should not cause significant hardship.

In some studies, they have shown having pernicious anemia increases the chances of developing stomach cancer.

Anemia of chronic disease

If the underlying condition that is causing anemia of chronic disease gets treated, the condition can resolve as a result.

Duration of Anemia

The duration of anemia depends on the type.

Iron deficiency anemia

Iron supplements (prescribed by your physician or hematologist) taken orally can work within 3 to 10 days to increase the body's production of red blood cells; however, it typically takes months to bring iron levels back to normal.

Aplastic anemia

When aplastic anemia is caused by radiation, chemotherapy, and other drugs, the condition tends to subside once treatments stop.

For women who develop aplastic anemia when pregnant, the condition usually improves once they're no longer pregnant.

Sickle cell anemia

Having sickle cell anemia means having a lifelong condition because a blood and bone marrow transplant are the only cure, and a small percentage of people with the disease actually get the transplant.

Pernicious anemia

While pernicious anemia is a lifelong condition, treatment can help people feel well and live normal lives. In most cases, early diagnosis and treatment can help reverse complications of pernicious anemia, such as nerve damage.

Anemia of chronic disease

When the underlying condition that is causing anemia of chronic disease is treated, the condition tends to go away.

Treatments and Medication Options for Anemia

Each type of anemia will require a different type of treatment.

Medication Options

Growth factors, both naturally occurring and man-made, are hormones that stimulate bone marrow to make blood cells to treat aplastic anemia. Immunosuppressive drug therapy is another option.

Severe iron-deficiency anemia may require intravenous (IV) iron therapy, blood transfusion, or injections of the synthetic hormone erythropoietin, which is normally produced by the kidneys.

When successful, a bone marrow transplant or stem cell transplant may cure sickle cell anemia.

B12 supplements or shots may help pernicious anemia.

Chemotherapy or bone marrow transplantation may be needed for anemias associated with bone marrow disease.

Oxygen, pain relievers, and oral and intravenous fluids can help reduce pain and prevent complications in sickle cell anemia.

Alternative and Complementary Therapies

When low iron is caused by an inadequate diet lacking iron-rich foods, a focus on high-iron foods such as meat, poultry, fish, beans, tofu, dried fruits, dark green leafy vegetables, and iron-fortified foods like breads and cereals can help.

Eating or drinking foods and drinks high in vitamin C, such as orange juice, broccoli, peppers, and more, can help your body absorb iron when you eat it.

In some instances, iron-deficiency anemia can be prevented with the following methods:

- Treating blood loss For those with heavy menstrual periods or stomach issues, such as fre uent diarrhea or blood in your stool, addressing the root imbalances leading to blood loss can help prevent anemia.

- Consuming foods with iron Eating foods with high levels of iron, such as lean meat, chicken, dark leafy vegetables, and beans can increase iron levels.

- Ensuring enough vitamin C Drinks and foods with vitamin C like orange juice, strawberries, and broccoli can help the body absorb iron.

- A balanced diet Balanced diets can ensure enough iron is being consumed.

- Limiting coffee or tea with meals If you drink coffee and tea with meals, they can make it difficult for your body to absorb iron.
- Caution with calcium pills Because calcium can affect how your body absorbs iron, ask your doctor what the best approach is for getting both enough calcium and enough iron.

While there's no known prevention for aplastic anemia, staying clear of insecticides, herbicides, organic solvents, paint removers, and other toxic chemicals may lower your risk.

While pernicious anemia caused by a lack of intrinsic factor is not preventable, those who develop the disease because they lack B12 in their diet can potentially reduce the impact by eating foods high in B12, such as beef, eggs, fortified cereal, and more, yet ultimately they are likely to need high-dose B12

supplementation or injections under their doctors'
guidance.

When anemia is not treated, it can cause complications, including:

- Extreme fatigue resulting in the inability to function.
- Pregnancy complications, including premature birth.
- Heart problems, such as irregular heartbeat, enlarged heart, and heart failure.
- Death caused by loss of blood with sickle cell anemia.

Research and Statistics: Who Has Anemia?

Anemia affects 1.62 billion people worldwide, and disproportionately occurs in countries with limited resources, according to the WHO. Children who are preschool age are greatly affected. Nonpregnant women have the greatest prevalence, while men experience the lowest occurrences. As the most common blood condition in the United States, anemia affects three million Americans.

Related Conditions and Causes of Anemia

In some cases, B12 deficiency can be caused by conditions such as infections, surgery, medicines, and diet.

Crohn's and celiac disease can also interfere with B12 absorption.

Anemia of chronic disease can be caused by inflammatory diseases, such as rheumatoid arthritis, ulcerative colitis, Crohn's disease, inflammatory bowel disease, lupus, diabetes, and degenerative joint disease.

Infectious diseases, such as HIV, hepatitis, tuberculosis, heart infection, and bone infection, can also lead to anemia of chronic disease.

Additionally, kidney failure and cancers, such as Hodgkin disease, non-Hodgkin lymphoma, and lung and breast cancer, can cause anemia.

Iron-Deficiency Anemia Quiz

Sometimes getting the right amount of iron from your diet isn't enough if your body isn't able to absorb it properly. For instance, people who've had intestinal surgery, such as gastric bypass, or those with Crohn's disease or celiac disease, may have trouble absorbing iron. Iron absorption can also be limited by prescription medicines that reduce acid in the stomach.

Blood loss is another cause of iron deficiency anemia because whenever you lose blood from your body, iron loss also occurs. If you don't have enough iron stored in your body to make up for the iron lost in your blood, you can develop anemia.

Blood loss that leads to low iron levels can result from:

- Heavy menstrual periods
- Bleeding fibroids (noncancerous growths) in the uterus
- Childbirth
- Internal bleeding caused by an ulcer, colon polyp, colon cancer, urinary tract bleeding, or use of pain medications
- Injuries or surgery
- Repeated blood drawings

Symptoms of iron-deficiency anemia vary depending on how severe your anemia is. If you have mild to moderate iron-deficiency anemia, you may not have any signs or symptoms. But as the condition worsens, you may experience:

- Fatigue
- Pale skin

- Weakness

- Shortness of breath

- Chest pain

- Frequent infections

- Headache

- Dizziness or light-headedness

- Cold hands and feet

- Swelling or soreness of your tongue

- Cracks around your mouth

- Brittle nails

- Fast heartbeat

- Poor appetite

- Restless legs syndrome

- Enlarged spleen

- Cravings for nonfood items, such as ice, dirt, paint, or starch

If you're mildly anemic, your doctor may recommend a diet filled with iron-rich foods. The foods with the highest iron content are:

- Meat, especially beef and liver
- Poultry — chicken livers are packed with iron
- Fish and shellfish, especially oysters
- Leafy greens, like kale, spinach, and broccoli
- Beans and peas
- Iron-enriched breads, pastas, and cereals

Take note that iron from vegetable sources is less readily absorbed than iron from meat, poultry, or seafood.

Anemia Resources

With all forms of anemia, tiredness or fatigue is the most common symptom because of low red blood cell count. Shortness of breath, dizziness, headache, coldness in your hands and feet, pale or yellowish skin, and chest pain are other signs.

When you have low red blood cells, your heart has to work harder to move oxygen-rich blood through your body. When this occurs, you can experience irregular heartbeat, enlarged heart, or even heart failure.

If your doctor suspects you may have pernicious anemia, he or she can confirm it with blood tests. Bone marrow tests can also detect this type of anemia because when pernicious anemia is present, bone marrow cells that turn into blood cells are larger than normal.

You can treat anemia symptoms naturally in the following ways:

Nourish Your Spleen

The first natural treatment for anemia is really nourishing your spleen. Your spleen is an organ that is responsible for red blood cell production, as well as keeping fluids together in your system. If your spleen isn't healthy, that's one of the first factors that's going to cause anemia.

There are specific foods that will actually help nourish your spleen, helping you overcome anemia symptoms naturally. That first food group is squash, specifically pumpkin, acorn s uash, butternut s uash, spaghetti s uash and those bright orange-colored foods. Think fall harvest! Those sorts of foods are fantastic for nourishing the spleen. Aim for getting one to two servings of squash in your daily diet. If you want some ideas, try my Butternut Squash Soup as a starter.

The other food group that's very important for nourishing your spleen and red blood cell production is green leafy vegetables like nutrition-rich spinach, kale and chard. Having one serving of those per day, something like a Kale Caesar Salad or sautéed spinach, is also very nourishing to your spleen.

Last, but not least, bitter foods are great for the spleen, specifically vegetables like romaine lettuce and arugula salad. You can even consume bitter herbs before a meal as a supplement. But anything that's sort of a bitter food is very nourishing for the spleen.

Use Probiotics for a Healthy Gut

Step number two to help you naturally overcome anemia symptoms is to boost gut health with probiotics. Gut health is crucial for absorption of nutrients. The principle is not: "You are what you eat." Rather, it is: "You are what you digest." If you're not digesting properly and absorbing and assimilating nutrients properly, you're not absorbing iron!

For a lot of people taking iron supplements, unfortunately they might not be working all that well. The reason is that their digestive system isn't healthy; they probably have a condition called leaky gut syndrome. Leaky gut doesn't allow you to properly absorb iron as well as certain other vitamins and minerals, like vitamin B12, magnesium and zinc.

A medical study out of Stanford found that when somebody supplements with probiotics, all of their B vitamin levels tend to go up, along with iron levels. So rather than simply popping an iron tablet without fixing the underlying problem, try to make changes that tackle the root problem of poor gut health. I recommend you add in probiotic-rich foods to your diet like real homemade yogurt, goat milk kefir and sauerkraut. Then taking a probiotic supplement, typically 50 billion to 100 billion IUs daily, can definitely help support your iron absorption.

Consume Iron-Rich Foods

The next step in helping you overcome anemia symptoms is consuming iron-rich foods. The richest sources of heme iron (the more absorbable form) in the diet include lean meat and seafood. Dietary sources of non-heme iron include nuts, beans, vegetables and fortified grain products. In the United States, about half of dietary iron comes from bread, cereal and other grain products, but I recommend focusing on healthier options that are easier to digest instead.

Some of the best iron foods include beef liver and chicken liver. Liver? It might sound gross to you, but if you buy organic chicken liver at your local farmers' market or at your health food store, you can put it in a slow cooker with chicken in e ual ratios, or about a third liver, two-thirds chicken. Include vegetables like carrots, celery, onions and sea salt. This is the perfect meal to help replenish your liver, as it's very high in iron. For other iron-rich foods, look toward organic, grass-fed meats like beef, bison and lamb. Also, eat spinach, kale and chard. Have a bison burger with a side of spinach, which is fantastic for helping you to reverse anemia.

Reduce Stress

If you're emotionally stressed out and you struggle with forgiveness, anger, or have chronic worry and anxiety, those things really deplete your spleen and your liver and will exhaust those organs. So, really make sure that you are scheduling in times of relaxation and fun during your week. Plus, get plenty of sleep at night. Those things will really help recharge your system and body and help you relieve stress. If you do those things, you're going to see fantastic results in overcoming anemia.

Consider Taking Supplements

In addition to making the holistic changes described above, you can likely benefit from taking a B vitamin complex supplement that includes folate (not folic acid!), as well as an iron supplement, according to the NHLBI.

Another bonus tip related to stress and spleen health: In Chinese medicine, anemia is very closely related to the spleen. And, certain herbs actually help support the spleen, especially ginseng. Ginseng is known as an adaptogenic herb that lowers cortisol. It can help your body better deal with stress. Lastly, benefit-rich beets also help with a healthy circulatory system and healthy iron levels.

8 Types Of Food That Can Help You Fight Anaemia!

Anaemia happens when the body lacks enough healthy red blood cells. As a result, the blood becomes incapable of carrying an ade uate amount of oxygen. Anaemia can be temporary or long term and can range from mild to severe.

Do you Feel Fatigued All the Time?

Fatigue is one of the most defining symptoms of anaemia. If anaemia is caused due to a chronic disease, it can mask the signs of anaemia making it challenging to detect. Depending on the cause of anaemia, there might or might not be symptoms. If there are, they will be:

- Weakness

- Irregular heartbeats

- Dizziness or lightheadedness

- Cold hands and feet

- Pale or yellowish skin

- Shortness of breath

- Chest pain

- Headaches

A diet plan with iron-rich foods can help control if not cure anaemia completely. Without enough iron, our body cannot make enough haemoglobin. That becomes a big problem because haemoglobin is the substance in red blood cells that carries oxygen from the heart to the body tissues. About 50% of pregnant women, 20% of women, and 3% of men lack enough iron in their bodies.

Foods for Anaemia

Most anaemic patients are advised to take 150 to 200 milligrams of iron every day. Make sure to have these foods to fight anaemia:

1) Fruits and Vegetables

- Curly kale and other varieties
- Collard greens
- Pomegranates
- Swiss chard
- Red and yellow peppers
- Watercress
- Spinach
- Dandelion greens
- Oranges
- Strawberries
- Lemon

- Key lime
- Sweet potatoes
- Beet greens

Dark leafy greens like spinach are a great source of non-heme iron. Vitamin C from citrus fruits helps the stomach to absorb iron. Swiss chard and Collard greens are good sources of both Vitamin C and iron.

2) Nuts and Seeds

- Cashews
- Hemp seeds
- Sunflower seeds
- Pumpkin seeds
- Pistachios
- Pine nuts
- Walnuts
- Peanuts

- Almonds

- Hazelnut

Nuts and seeds are some of the most nutrient-dense foods. One ounce of pistachios can provide 6.1% of the re uired daily value of iron in a person.

3) Meat and Fish

- Lamb

- Liver

- Oysters

- Salmon

- Perch

- Beef

- Venison

- Shellfish

- Shrimp

- Tuna

- Halibut

- Haddock

- Chicken

Meat and fish have heme iron. Lean cut white meat like chicken is a great source of heme protein. Three ounces of grilled chicken with sides of broccoli, sauteed spinach, and tomatoes can make for a great iron-rich meal for people suffering from anaemia.

4) Eggs

Eggs are known for their proteins, but they also pack a high level of iron. Eggs can be had paired with whole-grain toast, lightly roasted tomatoes, and uinoa for breakfast that will provide a great start to the day.

5) Beans and Pulses

- Chickpeas

- Black-eyed peas

- Black beans

- Lima beans

- Kidney beans

- Soybeans

  Lentils are supposed to be a superfood for anaemic patients. Half a cup of lentils has about 3.3 milligrams of iron, which is around 20% of what your body needs throughout the day. Beans and pulses work for both vegetarians and meat-eaters and provide a good amount of iron.

6) Blackstrap Molasses

Blackstrap molasses are loaded with iron. They are a total nutritional powerhouse because of calcium, Vitamin B6, selenium, and magnesium. They are perfect for anaemic patients because apart from providing the iron they desperately need, blackstrap molasses also keep them healthy due to the presence of other integral nutrients.

7) Grains

Iron-fortified pasta, cereals, and grains are good options for getting the much-needed iron. However, there are natural options too. They are all rich in iron and can help in shooting up the haemoglobin level in blood.

- Quinoa
- Oats

- Whole wheat

- Kamut

- Teff

8) Fortified Food

There are different types of food that are fortified with iron. You can add these to your diet if you are a vegetarian or cannot keep down other sources of iron.

- Fortified, ready-to-eat cereals

- Fortified pasta

- Fortified white rice

- Fortified orange juice

- Foods made from fortified white flour, like bread

- Foods made from fortified cornmeal

Foods to Avoid if You Are Anaemic

Some types of food interfere with the absorption of iron. As a result, having all that iron-rich food sometimes might prove to be redundant if had with these foods:

- Yoghurt
- Raw milk
- Cheese
- Sardines
- Broccoli
- Tofu
- Tea and coffee
- Food containing tannins like corn, grapes, sorghum

How Can You Get More Iron From Your Diet?

- Have food rich in iron
- Include food in your diet that will help you absorb the iron
- Cook food in a cast-iron skillet
- Cook food for shorter periods
- Refrain from drinking tea or coffee with meals
- Consult with your doctor and choose supplements containing ferrous salts

How Does Your Body use Iron From Iron-Rich Foods?

The iron from iron-rich foods is absorbed through the upper part of the small intestine. Dietary iron is of two types: heme iron and non-heme iron. Heme iron is derived from haemoglobin. Our body absorbs iron mostly from heme sources. Heme iron can be found in fish, red meats, and poultry. Non-heme iron is mainly found in plant sources. Meat, seafood, and chicken, however, contain a little bit of both.

Following dosage instructions is essential because an excess of iron can cause iron toxicity. Consult with your doctor, go to a dietician if re uired and get yourself a proper diet chart. No one food can cure anaemia, but the right diet can help a lot. Follow it well, and anaemia shouldn't pose to be a problem anymore.

Diet to Help Reduce Anemia

Even though anemia is so common, it's possible for most healthy people without serious illnesses to prevent anemia by eating a healthy, unprocessed diet. Above you read about foods to avoid in order to manage anemia symptoms and also candida. Now here are some of the best foods to include in your diet in order to overcome anemia:

- Liver: Beef liver is very high in iron and vitamin B12 and a variety of other important minerals. If unable to consume cow liver, make sure you include grass-fed, organic beef as an alternative.
- Brewer's yeast: High in folic acid, vitamin 12, and iron. Add to cereal, salad or juice.
- Foods high in vitamin C: Vitamin C helps with iron absorption. If you are eating a high-iron food (beef) try to include a source of vitamin C at that same meal such as tomatoes, peppers or strawberries.
- Green leafy vegetables: These provide a significant amount of iron and folic acid. Raw spinach is high in oxalic acid, which can reduce iron absorption; however, steaming spinach

will reduce this acid. Other green leafy vegetables to include are steamed kale and broccoli.

- Natural sweeteners (in small amounts): If you're wondering what to do when you need to use some sort of sweetener but are avoiding added sugar, try blackstrap molasses or raw local honey in small amounts (about one tablespoon at most at a time). Blackstrap molasses can be taken in servings of about one spoonful daily, as it is very high in iron. Local honey or stevia are two other good options in terms of keeping too much sugar out of your diet, but lightly sweetening foods.

1. Mushroom & Tofu Stir-Fry

Ingredients

4 tablespoons peanut oil or canola oil, divided

1 pound mixed mushrooms, sliced

1 medium red bell pepper, diced

1 bunch scallions, trimmed and cut into 2-inch pieces

1 tablespoon grated fresh ginger

1 large clove garlic, grated

1 (8 ounce) container baked tofu or smoked tofu, diced

3 tablespoons oyster sauce or vegetarian oyster sauce (see Tip)

Directions

Heat 2 tablespoons oil in a large flat-bottom wok or cast-iron skillet over high heat. Add mushrooms and bell pepper; cook, stirring occasionally, until soft, about 4 minutes. Stir in scallions, ginger and garlic; cook for 30 seconds more. Transfer the vegetables to a bowl.

Add the remaining 2 tablespoons oil and tofu to the pan. Cook, turning once, until browned, 3 to 4 minutes. Stir in the vegetables and oyster sauce. Cook, stirring, until hot, about 1 minute.

2. Balsamic-Parmesan Sautéed Spinach

Ingredients

2 tablespoons extra-virgin olive oil

3 cloves garlic, minced

1 pound fresh spinach

¼ teaspoon salt

¼ teaspoon ground pepper

2 tablespoons grated Parmesan cheese

4 teaspoons good- uality balsamic vinegar or balsamic glaze

Instructions

Heat oil in a large pot over medium heat. Add garlic and cook, stirring, until fragrant, 30 seconds to 1 minute. Add spinach, salt and pepper; toss to coat. Cook, stirring, until just wilted, 3 to 5 minutes. Remove from heat and stir in Parmesan. Drizzle with vinegar (or glaze) and serve immediately.

3. Skillet Steak with Mushroom Sauce

Ingredients

12 ounces boneless beef top sirloin steak, cut 1 inch thick and trimmed

2 teaspoons salt-free steak grilling seasoning, such as Mrs. Dash®

2 teaspoons canola oil

6 ounces broccoli rabe, trimmed

2 cups frozen peas

3 cups sliced fresh mushrooms

1 cup unsalted beef broth

1 tablespoon whole-grain mustard

2 teaspoons cornstarch

¼ teaspoon salt

Directions

Preheat oven to 350 degrees F. Sprinkle meat with steak seasoning. In a 12-inch cast-iron skillet heat oil over medium-high. Add meat and broccoli rabe. Cook 4 minutes, turning broccoli rabe once (do not turn meat). Place peas around meat. Transfer skillet to oven and bake 8 minutes or until meat is medium-rare (145 degrees F). Remove meat and vegetables from skillet; cover and keep warm.

For sauce, add mushrooms to drippings in skillet. Cook over medium-high 3 minutes, stirring occasionally. Whisk together the beef broth, mustard, cornstarch and salt; stir into mushrooms. Cook and stir until thick and bubbly. Cook and stir 1 minute more. Serve meat and vegetables with sauce.

4. Eggplant & Chickpea Baked Pasta

Ingredients

8 ounces whole-wheat fusilli

½ cup coarse dry whole-wheat breadcrumbs (see Note)

1 tablespoon extra-virgin olive oil

3 cups Eggplant & Chickpea Stew (see associated recipe)

1 cup crumbled feta cheese

½ cup chopped fresh mint or basil, divided

2 tablespoons lemon juice

Directions

Preheat oven to 350 degrees F. Coat an 8-inch-s uare (or similar 2- uart) baking dish with cooking spray.

Bring a large pot of water to a boil. Cook pasta according to package directions. Drain and rinse.

Combine breadcrumbs and oil in a small bowl. Toss the pasta with stew, feta, 1/4 cup mint (or basil) and lemon juice in a large bowl. Spread the mixture in the prepared baking dish. Top with the breadcrumb mixture.

Bake until the topping is golden and crispy, about 30 minutes. Sprinkle with the remaining 1/4 cup mint (or basil).

5. Sheet-Pan Steak & Potatoes

Ingredients

1 pound potatoes, cut into 1/2-inch wedges

2 tablespoons extra-virgin olive oil, divided

¾ teaspoon salt, divided

¾ teaspoon ground pepper, divided

4 cups chopped asparagus

1 ¼ pounds skirt steak, trimmed

½ teaspoon garlic powder

½ teaspoon dried rosemary

3 tablespoons crumbled blue cheese

Directions

Preheat oven to 425 degrees F.

Toss potatoes with 1 tablespoon oil and 1/4 teaspoon each salt and pepper in a large bowl. Spread evenly on a rimmed baking sheet. Roast for 15 minutes.

Toss asparagus with the remaining 1 tablespoon oil and 1/4 teaspoon each salt and pepper in the bowl. Stir into the potatoes on the baking sheet.

Sprinkle steak with garlic powder, rosemary and the remaining 1/4 teaspoon each salt and pepper. Place on top of the vegetables. Roast until the steak is cooked and the vegetables are tender, 10 to 15 minutes more.

Transfer the steak to a serving platter. Stir blue cheese into the vegetables and serve with the steak.

6. Tofu, Mushroom & Bok Choy Soba Noodle Bowls

Ingredients

3 tablespoons canola oil, divided

2 teaspoons toasted sesame oil

1 teaspoon grated fresh ginger

2 cloves garlic, grated

4 scallions, sliced, greens and whites separated, divided

1 serrano pepper, thinly sliced

4 cups low-sodium no-chicken broth (see Tip)

2 tablespoons reduced-sodium tamari or soy sauce (see Tip)

2 heads baby bok choy, thinly sliced

5 ounces sliced shiitake mushroom caps

¼ teaspoon salt

8 ounces buckwheat soba or udon noodles

1 (14 ounce) package extra-firm tofu, drained and cut into bite-size cubes

Fresh cilantro for garnish

Directions

Bring a medium saucepan of water to a boil.

Heat 1 tablespoon canola oil in a large saucepan over medium heat. Add sesame oil, ginger, garlic, scallion whites and serrano and cook until fragrant, about 1 minute. Add broth and tamari (or soy sauce) and bring to a boil. Cover and simmer while you prepare vegetables and noodles.

Heat the remaining 2 tablespoons canola oil in a large skillet or flat-bottom wok over high heat. Add bok choy and shiitakes and cook, stirring occasionally, until well browned, about 8 minutes. Sprinkle with salt. Remove from heat.

Cook noodles in the boiling water according to package directions. Drain and divide among 4 serving bowls. Top with the vegetables and tofu and ladle on the hot broth. Top with scallion greens and garnish with cilantro, if desired.

7. Kale & Quinoa Salad with Lemon Dressing

Ingredients

1 bunch lacinato kale, stemmed and chopped

6 tablespoons extra-virgin olive oil

3 tablespoons lemon juice

2 tablespoons chopped shallot

1 teaspoon honey

½ teaspoon salt

¼ teaspoon ground pepper

2 cups grape or cherry tomatoes, halved

2 cups cooked uinoa

1 English cucumber, thinly sliced

1 medium red bell pepper, sliced

1 medium yellow bell pepper, sliced

1 (15 ounce) can unsalted chickpeas, rinsed

¾ cup feta cheese, crumbled

½ cup sliced almonds, toasted

Disrections

Place kale in a large serving bowl. Whisk together oil, lemon juice, shallot, honey, salt and pepper in a small bowl. Pour 2 to 3 tablespoons of the dressing over the kale; lightly massage until slightly wilted, 1 to 2 minutes.

Top the kale with tomatoes, uinoa, cucumber, peppers, chickpeas, feta and almonds. Drizzle with the remaining dressing and toss before serving.

8. Lentil & Goat Cheese Toast

Ingredients

2 tablespoons goat cheese

2 slices olive sourdough bread, toasted

.666 cup rinsed canned French green lentils

2 tablespoons chopped walnuts, toasted

Directions

Spread 1 tablespoon goat cheese on each slice of toast. Top each with 1/3 cup lentils and 1 tablespoon walnuts.

9. Vegetarian Potato-Kale Soup

Ingredients

1 tablespoon extra-virgin olive oil

1 small sweet onion, halved and thinly sliced

3 cloves garlic, finely chopped

4 cups low-sodium vegetable broth

2 cups water

1 pound baby red potatoes, halved lengthwise

2 medium parsnips, peeled and sliced 1/4-inch thick

1 teaspoon chopped fresh rosemary, plus more
for garnish

¼ teaspoon salt

1 small bunch lacinato kale, stemmed and
chopped

½ cup grated Parmesan cheese, plus more for
garnish

¼ cup heavy cream

1 tablespoon lemon juice

Directions

Heat oil in a Dutch oven or large heavy pot over
medium-high heat. Add onion; cook, stirring
occasionally, under tender, about 5 minutes.
Add garlic; cook, stirring constantly, until
fragrant, about 30 seconds. Stir in broth, water,
potatoes, parsnips, rosemary and salt; bring to
a boil. Reduce heat to medium-low; cover and
cook, stirring occasionally, until the vegetables

are tender, about 15 minutes. Using the back of a spoon, gently mash the vegetables to slightly thicken the soup.

Stir in kale, Parmesan and cream; cook over medium-low heat, stirring occasionally, until the kale is wilted, about 10 minutes more. Stir in lemon juice just before serving. Garnish with additional rosemary and Parmesan, if desired.

10. Pan-Seared Steak with Crispy Herbs & Escarole

Ingredients

1 pound sirloin steak, about 1/2 inch thick

½ teaspoon salt, divided

½ teaspoon ground pepper, divided

2 tablespoons grapeseed oil or canola oil

4 cloves garlic, crushed

5 sprigs fresh thyme

3 sprigs fresh sage

1 sprig fresh rosemary

16 cups chopped escarole (about 1 pound)

Directions

Sprinkle steak with 1/4 teaspoon each salt and pepper. Heat a large cast-iron skillet over medium-high heat. Add the steak and cook until charred on one side, about 3 minutes. Turn the steak over and add oil, garlic, thyme, sage and rosemary. Cook, stirring the herbs occasionally, until an instant-read thermometer inserted in the thickest part of the steak reaches 125 degrees F for medium-rare, 3 to 4 minutes. Transfer the steak to a plate and top with the garlic and herbs. Tent with foil.

Add escarole and the remaining 1/4 teaspoon each salt and pepper to the pan. Cook, stirring often, until the escarole starts to wilt, about 2 minutes. Thinly slice the steak and serve with the escarole and crispy herbs.

11. Steaks with goulash sauce & sweet potato fries

Ingredients

3 tsp rapeseed oil , plus extra for the steaks

250g sweet potatoes , peeled and cut into narrow chips

1 tbsp fresh thyme leaves

2 small onions , halved and sliced (190g)

1 green pepper , deseeded and diced

2 garlic cloves , sliced

1 tsp smoked paprika

85g cherry tomatoes , halved

1 tbsp tomato purée

1 tsp vegetable bouillon powder

2 x 125g fillet steaks , rubbed with a little rapeseed oil

200g bag baby spinach , wilted in a pan or the microwave

Method

Heat oven to 240C/220C fan/gas 7 and put a wire rack on top of a baking tray. Toss the sweet potatoes and thyme with 2 tsp oil in a bowl, then scatter them over the rack and set aside until ready to cook.

Heat 1 tsp oil in a non-stick pan, add the onions, cover the pan and leave to cook for 5 mins. Take off the lid and stir – they should be a little charred now. Stir in the green pepper and garlic, cover the pan and cook for 5 mins more. Put the potatoes in the oven and bake for 15 mins.

While the potatoes are cooking, stir the paprika into the onions and peppers, pour in 150ml water and stir in the cherry tomatoes, tomato purée and bouillon. Cover and simmer for 10 mins.

Pan-fry the steak in a hot, non-stick pan for 2-3 mins each side depending on their thickness. Rest for 5 mins. Spoon the goulash sauce onto plates and top with the beef. Serve the chips and spinach alongside.

12. Rosemary balsamic lamb with vegetable mash

92

Ingredients

320g celeriac , peeled and diced

320g swede , peeled and diced

320g potato , peeled and diced

1 tbsp rapeseed oil

3 red onions , thinly sliced

550g lean, trimmed lamb steak , diced

1 tsp finely chopped rosemary

1 tbsp vegetable bouillon powder

2 tbsp balsamic vinegar

1 tbsp chopped parsley

320g spinach , to serve

320g frozen peas , to serve

Method

Put the celeriac, swede and potato in a large steamer, then steam for 25 mins until softened.

Meanwhile, heat the oil in a large non-stick frying pan and fry the onions for 10 mins until softened and golden. Push to the side of the pan, then add the lamb and rosemary and stir-fry over the heat until browned, but still a little pink in the middle – try not to overcook it as it will become tough and will need a longer cook to become tender again. Add the bouillon and balsamic vinegar with 200ml boiling water. Stir to make a sauce.

ash the steamed veg and spoon half into the centre of two plates. Top with half the lamb and gravy, scatter with the parsley and serve with the spinach and peas. Chill the remaining lamb and veg to reheat and serve on another evening.

13. Tofu & spinach cannelloni

Ingredients

2 tbsp olive oil

1 onion , chopped

3 garlic cloves , finely chopped

2 x 400g cans chopped tomatoes

50g pine nuts , roughly chopped

400g bag spinach

pinch grated nutmeg

349g pack silken tofu

300g pack fresh lasagne sheets

4 tbsp fresh breadcrumbs

Method

Heat half the oil in a pan, add onion and 1/3 of the garlic and fry for 4 mins until softened. Pour in tomatoes, season and bring to the boil. Reduce heat and cook for 10 mins until sauce thickens.

Heat half remaining oil in a frying pan and cook another 1/3 of garlic for 1 min, then add half the pine nuts and the spinach. Wilt spinach, then tip out excess li uid. Whizz tofu in a food processor or with a hand blender until smooth, then stir through the spinach with the nutmeg and some pepper. Remove from the heat; allow to cool slightly.

Heat oven to 200C/180C fan/gas 6. Pour half tomato sauce into a 20 x 30cm dish. Divide spinach mix between lasagne sheets, roll up and lay on top of sauce. Pour over remaining sauce. Bake for 30 mins.

Mix crumbs with remaining garlic and pine nuts. Sprinkle over top of dish, drizzle with remaining oil and bake for 10 mins until crumbs are golden.

14. Zingy teriyaki beef skewers

Ingredients

1 tbsp tamari or soy sauce

3 tbsp freshly s ueezed orange juice

15g chunk ginger , peeled and very finely
grated

2 garlic cloves , crushed

1 tsp honey (preferably raw)

¼ tsp chilli flakes

300g beef sirloin steak , trimmed of hard fat
and cut into long, thin strips

For the salad

100g long-grain brown rice

⅓ cucumber , cut into small cubes

2 medium carrots , peeled and sliced into
ribbons with a peeler

4 spring onions , trimmed and diagonally sliced

100g radishes , trimmed and sliced

20g coriander , leaves roughly chopped, plus extra to garnish

10g mint leaves , plus extra to garnish

1 tbsp cold-pressed rapeseed oil

zest and juice 1 lime

25g unsalted cashew nuts , toasted and roughly chopped

Method

Put the tamari, orange juice, ginger, garlic, honey and chilli flakes in a small saucepan with 100ml cold water and bring to the boil. Cook for 3-5 mins, boiling hard until well reduced, glossy and slightly syrupy. Remove from the heat, pour into a shallow dish and leave to cool.

Thread the beef onto 4 soaked wooden or metal skewers. Place in the marinade, turn and brush until well coated. Cover with cling film and marinate for 30 mins.

While the beef is marinating, prepare the salad. Half-fill a medium pan with water and bring to the boil. Cook the rice for about 20 mins or following pack instructions until tender. Rinse in a sieve under running water until cold, then drain well. Tip into a large bowl.

Add the cucumber, carrots, spring onions, radishes, coriander, mint, oil, lime zest and juice, and toss well together well. Season with a little black pepper. Divide between two plates and top with a sprinkling of nuts and extra herbs to garnish.

Heat the grill to high. (You could also cook the skewers on a non-stick griddle pan.) Put the skewers on a rack above a foil-lined baking tray, reserving any excess marinade. Grill the skewers close to the heat for 3-5 mins each side or until done to your liking. Brush with more marinade when they are turned. They should look sticky and glossy when cooked. Serve hot or cold with the rice salad.

15. Spinach, sweet potato & lentil dhal

Ingredients

1 tbsp sesame oil

1 red onion, finely chopped

1 garlic clove, crushed

thumb-sized piece ginger, peeled and finely chopped

1 red chilli, finely chopped

1½ tsp ground turmeric

1½ tsp ground cumin

2 sweet potatoes (about 400g/14oz), cut into even chunks

250g red split lentils

600ml vegetable stock

80g bag of spinach

4 spring onions, sliced on the diagonal, to serve

½ small pack of Thai basil, leaves torn, to serve

Method

Heat 1 tbsp sesame oil in a wide-based pan with a tight-fitting lid.

Add 1 finely chopped red onion and cook over a low heat for 10 mins, stirring occasionally, until softened.

Add 1 crushed garlic clove, a finely chopped thumb-sized piece of ginger and 1 finely chopped red chilli, cook for 1 min, then add 1½ tsp ground turmeric and 1½ tsp ground cumin and cook for 1 min more.

Turn up the heat to medium, add 2 sweet potatoes, cut into even chunks, and stir everything together so the potato is coated in the spice mixture.

Tip in 250g red split lentils, 600ml vegetable stock and some seasoning.

Bring the liquid to the boil, then reduce the heat, cover and cook for 20 mins until the lentils are tender and the potato is just holding its shape.

Taste and adjust the seasoning, then gently stir in the 80g spinach. Once wilted, top with the 4 diagonally sliced spring onions and ½ small pack torn basil leaves to serve.

Alternatively, allow to cool completely, then divide between airtight containers and store in the fridge for a healthy lunchbox.

16. Hearty lentil one pot

Ingredients

40g dried porcini mushrooms , roughly chopped

200g dried brown lentils

1 ½ tbsp chopped rosemary

3 tbsp rapeseed oil

2 large onions , roughly chopped

150g chestnut baby button mushrooms

4 garlic cloves , finely grated

2 tbsp vegetable bouillon powder

2 large carrots (350g), cut into chunks

3 celery sticks (165g), chopped

500g potatoes , cut into chunks

200g cavolo nero , shredded

Method

Cover the mushrooms in boiling water and leave to soak for 10 mins. Boil the lentils in a pan with plenty of water for 10 mins. Drain and rinse, then tip into a pan with the dried mushrooms and soaking water (don't add the last bit of the li uid as it can contain some grit), rosemary and 2 litres water. Season, cover and simmer for 20 mins.

Meanwhile, heat the oil in a large pan and fry the onions for 5 mins. Stir in the fresh mushrooms and garlic and fry for 5 mins more. Stir in the lentil mixture and bouillon powder, then add the carrots, celery and potatoes. Cover and cook for 20 mins, stirring often, until the veg and lentils are tender, topping up the water level if needed.

Remove any tough stalks from the cavolo nero, then add to the pan and cover and cook for 5 mins more. If you're following our Healthy Diet Plan, serve half in bowls, then chill the rest to eat another day. Will keep in the fridge for two to three days. Reheat in a pan until hot.

17. Mussels with chorizo, beans & cavolo nero

Ingredients

2 shallots , finely chopped

small bunch parsley , stalks and leaves separated and chopped

2 garlic cloves , finely chopped

100g cooking chorizo , skin removed and chopped

1 tbsp olive oil

100g cavolo nero , stems discarded, leaves shredded

150ml white wine or sherry

400g can cannellini beans , drained and rinsed

500g mussels , cleaned and beards removed

1 lemon , halved

Method

Gently cook the shallots, parsley stalks, garlic and chorizo in the oil in a large pan with a lid or casserole dish until the shallots are softened – about 5 mins. Add the cavolo nero and cook for a couple more mins, then add the wine and cook for another 1 min.

Stir in the beans, then add the mussels, ensuring they're well coated with the sauce, and cover with the lid. Cook for a few mins, shaking the pan to release the mussel juices, until they've all opened (discard any that haven't). Scatter over the parsley leaves and s ueeze over the lemon to serve.

18. Lamb & s uash biryani with cucumber raita

Ingredients

4 lean lamb steaks (about 400g), trimmed of all

fat, cut into chunks

2 garlic cloves , finely grated

8 tsp chopped fresh ginger

3 tsp ground coriander

4 tsp rapeseed oil

4 onions , sliced

2 red chillies , deseeded and chopped

170g brown basmati rice

320g diced butternut s uash

2 tsp cumin seeds

2 tsp vegetable bouillon powder

20cm length cucumber , grated

100ml bio yogurt

4 tbsp chopped mint , plus a few extra leaves

handful coriander , chopped

Method

Mix the lamb with the garlic, 2 tsp chopped ginger and 1 tsp ground coriander and set aside.

Heat 2 tsp oil in a non-stick pan. Add the onions, the remaining ginger and chilli and stir-fry briefly over a high heat so they start to soften. Add the rice and squash and stir over the heat for a few mins. Tip in all the remaining spices, then stir in 500ml boiling water and the bouillon. Cover the pan and simmer for 20 mins.

Meanwhile, mix the cucumber, yogurt and mint together in a bowl to make a raita. Chill half for later.

About 5 mins before the rice is ready, heat the remaining oil in a non-stick frying pan, add the lamb and stir for a few mins until browned but still nice tender. Toss into the spiced rice with the coriander and serve with the raita and a few mint or coriander leaves on top.

19. Slow-cooker beef stew

Ingredients

1 onion, chopped

2 celery sticks, finely chopped

2 tbsp rapeseed oil

3 carrots, halved and cut into chunks

2 bay leaves

½ pack thyme

2 tbsp tomato purée

2 tbsp Worcestershire sauce

2 beef stock cubes or stock pots

900g beef for braising such as skirt, buy a whole piece and cut it yourself for bigger chunks or buy ready-diced

2 tsp cornflour (optional)

½ small bunch parsley, chopped

buttery mash, to serve (optional)

Method

Fry the onion and celery in 1 tbsp oil over a low heat until they start to soften – about 5 mins. Add the carrots, bay and thyme, fry for 2 mins, stir in the purée and Worcestershire sauce, add 600ml boiling water, stir and tip everything into a slow cooker. Crumble over the stock cubes or add the stock pots and stir, then season with pepper (don't add salt as the stock may be salty).

Clean out the frying pan and fry the beef in the remaining oil in batches until it is well browned, then tip each batch into the slow cooker. Cook on low for 8-10 hrs, or on high for 4 hrs.

If you want to thicken the gravy, mix the cornflour with a splash of cold water to make a paste, then stir in 2 tbsp of the li uid from the slow cooker. Tip back into the slow cooker, stir and cook for a further 30 mins on high. Stir in the parsley and season again to taste. Serve with mash, if you like. Leave to cool before freezing.

20. Oysters with chilli & ginger dressing

Ingredients

12 oysters , shucked (see method for tips on preparing your oysters)

For the sauce

1 garlic clove , minced

thumb-sized piece ginger , finely chopped

2 tbsp mirin

1 tbsp soy sauce

4 spring onions , finely sliced

1 red chilli , finely chopped

2 tbsp sesame oil

bunch chives , finely chopped, to serve

Method

Shuck your oysters if not already prepared. Watch our video guide.

To make the sauce, mix all the ingredients together in a small bowl. Drizzle the sauce over the oysters, then sprinkle with chopped chives and serve straight away.